Kidney Dialysis diet Cookbook for Seniors

Essential Recipes and Tips for Senior Dialysis Patients

Mike J Clack

Mike J Clack
Copyright © 2024 by

All rights reserved. No part of this publication may be reproduced, distributed, or transmitted in any form or by any means, including photocopying, recording, or other electronic or mechanical methods, without the prior written permission of the publisher.

Disclaimer:

The information provided in this book is for educational and informational purposes only. It is not intended as medical advice and should not be construed as such. The contents of this book are based on the author's research, experience, and opinions. Readers are encouraged to consult with healthcare professionals for personalized advice and recommendations regarding their specific health conditions and needs. The author and publisher disclaim any liability or responsibility for any adverse consequences resulting directly or indirectly from the use or application of the information contained in this book. Readers assume full responsibility for their actions and decisions based on the information contained herein.

How to Use This Book

We are pleased that Mike J. Clack's Kidney Dialysis Diet Cookbook for Seniors has been chosen. This book's objective is to provide practical advice and information to those undergoing dialysis and managing renal sickness. To get the most of this book, consider the following suggestions:

1. Read Carefully: Devote your whole attention to every chapter and section. Make a note of the key points, counsel, and recommendations shared.

2. Refer to Specific Sections: Use the index and table of contents to get information on specific topics or topics that pique your interest. You could navigate to the sections that now pertain to you based on your needs or interests.

3. Take Notes: Consider keeping a notebook or journal handy as you read. Any relevant thoughts, points, or questions that arise should be noted. This might help you understand and serve as a resource for you later on.

4. Put the Advice into Practice: Apply the strategies, directives, and recommendations found in the book to your daily tasks. Try a few different approaches to find which one works best for you.

5. Consult with Healthcare Professionals: This book provides a lot of information, but for suggestions and guidance tailored to your particular circumstances and health requirements, you should consult with your healthcare team, which includes physicians, dietitians, and other experts.

6. Share with Others: If you find the information in this book to be enlightening and beneficial, consider sending it to family members, friends, or support groups who may find it beneficial.

7. Stay Inspired and engaged: To improve your health and well-being, stay motivated and engaged. Make questions, be informed, and never stop acquiring new skills to improve your life.

I hope everything is okay with you.

Clack, Mike J

TABLE OF CONTENTS

Mike J Clack
How to Use This Book
TABLE OF CONTENTS
Introduction
Overview of Kidney Disease
Types, Causes, and Symptoms of Kidney Disease
Symptoms and Signs of Kidney Dysfunction
Overview of Kidney Diseases
Types of Kidney Diseases:
Common Causes of Kidney Disease
Dietary Guidelines
Instructions for Following a Dialysis Diet

- Strategies for Complying with Dietary Limitations
- 30-Day Dialysis Diet Meal Plan
- Weekly Meal Plan Summary
- Daily Meal Plans with Recipes and Portion Calculations
- Recipes
- Meal Ideas for Breakfast
- Lunch Recipes
- 10 Dialysis Patient Breakfast Ideas
- Dinner Recipes
- 10 Lunch Ideas for Dialysis Patients
- Snack Recipes
- Easy and Nutritious Snack Ideas
- Kidney Health and Dialysis
- Hemodialysis
- Peritoneal Dialysis
- Function of Healthy Kidneys

Dietary Basics for Patients Receiving Dialysis
Value of a Balanced Diet
Foods to Restrict and Steer Clear of
Tips and Strategies for Meal Planning
Strategies for Successful Meal Planning
Buying Advice for Dialysis Friendly Foods
Special Considerations and Tips
Managing Nutritional Difficulties
Advice for Dialysis Patients When Dining Out
Guidelines for Physical Activity and Exercise
Strategies for Stress Management
Simple and Healthful Smoothie Ideas
Breakfast Smoothies Low in Potassium

Ideas for Nutrient-Dense Smoothies

Recipes for Breakfast Bowls for Patients on Dialysis

Conclusion

Summary of Important Ideas

Sources of Additional Information

Request for Review

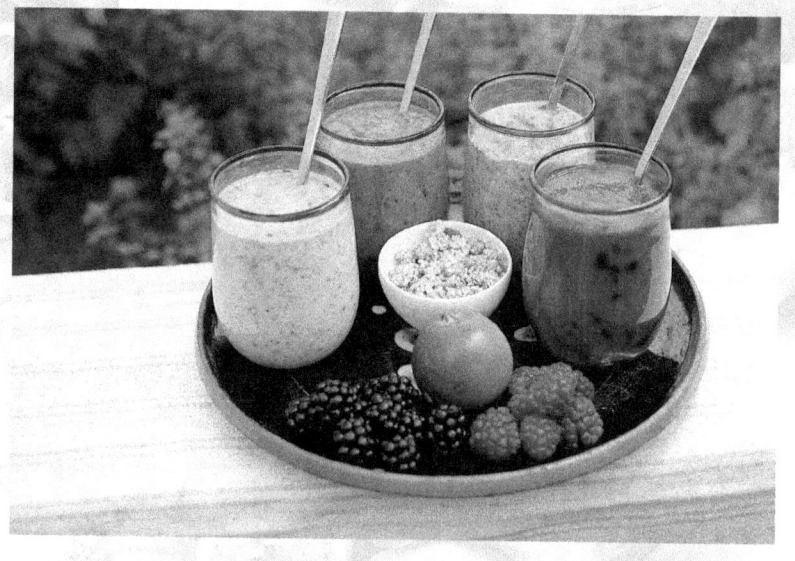

Introduction

Overview of Kidney Disease

Kidney disease, also known as renal disease or nephropathy, encompasses a range of conditions that affect the kidneys' ability to function properly. The kidneys play a crucial role in filtering waste products and excess fluids from the blood, regulating electrolyte levels, and producing hormones that help control blood pressure and stimulate red blood cell production.

There are various types of kidney disease, each with its own causes, symptoms, and treatment approaches. Some common types of kidney disease include:

Chronic Kidney Disease (CKD): This is a long-term condition characterized by gradual loss of kidney function over time. CKD can progress through five stages, with the final stage, known as end-stage renal disease (ESRD), requiring dialysis or kidney transplantation for survival.

Acute Kidney Injury (AKI): Also referred to as acute renal failure, AKI is a sudden and often reversible loss of kidney function, typically caused by factors such as dehydration, severe infection, or exposure to certain medications or toxins.

Polycystic Kidney Disease (PKD): PKD is an inherited disorder characterized by the growth of fluid-filled cysts in the kidneys, which can lead to kidney enlargement, high blood pressure, and kidney failure over time.

Glomerulonephritis: This refers to inflammation of the glomeruli, the tiny blood vessels in the kidneys responsible for filtering waste and excess fluid from the blood. Glomerulonephritis can be acute or chronic and may result from infections, autoimmune diseases, or other underlying conditions.

Diabetic Nephropathy: Diabetes is a leading cause of kidney disease, as high blood sugar levels can damage the kidneys' blood vessels and impair their function over time. Diabetic nephropathy is a common complication of both type 1 and type 2 diabetes.

Symptoms of kidney disease can vary depending on the type and severity of the condition but may include fatigue, swelling (edema), changes in urine output, blood in the urine, high blood pressure, nausea, and difficulty concentrating. Early detection and management of kidney disease are crucial for preserving kidney function and preventing complications.

Comprehending the Significance of Nutrition for Individuals Receiving Dialysis

Nutrition plays a crucial role in the overall health and well-being of individuals undergoing dialysis treatment for kidney failure. Dialysis is a life-saving procedure that helps remove waste products and excess fluid from the blood when the kidneys are no longer able to perform this function adequately. However, dialysis also leads to significant changes in the body's nutritional needs and metabolism, making proper nutrition essential for managing various aspects of health and optimizing treatment outcomes.

Dialysis helps remove excess fluid from the body, but individuals on dialysis still need to closely monitor their fluid intake to prevent fluid overload and related complications such as high blood pressure, swelling, and shortness of breath. Proper hydration and adherence to fluid restrictions prescribed by healthcare providers are essential.

The kidneys play a crucial role in regulating electrolyte levels in the body, including sodium, potassium, and phosphorus. Dialysis can disrupt this balance, leading to electrolyte imbalances that can affect heart function, muscle contractions, and nerve transmission. Following a kidney-friendly diet that limits high-potassium and high-phosphorus foods while ensuring adequate intake of essential nutrients is essential for maintaining electrolyte balance.

High blood pressure (hypertension) is a common complication of kidney failure and can further damage the kidneys and increase the risk of cardiovascular disease. A diet low in sodium and rich in fruits, vegetables, and whole grains can help lower blood pressure and reduce the risk of complications.

Individuals undergoing dialysis are at increased risk of malnutrition due to factors such as decreased appetite, dietary restrictions, and loss of nutrients during dialysis treatments. Consuming adequate protein and calories is essential for preserving muscle mass, preventing weight loss, and supporting overall health.

Chronic kidney disease can lead to abnormalities in bone metabolism, including decreased bone density and an increased risk of fractures. A balanced diet that includes sufficient calcium and vitamin D is essential for maintaining bone health and preventing conditions such as renal osteodystrophy.

Proper nutrition is essential for supporting the immune system, promoting wound healing, and reducing the risk of complications associated with kidney disease and dialysis, such as infections, cardiovascular disease, and impaired cognitive function.

Types, Causes, and Symptoms of Kidney Disease

Symptoms and Signs of Kidney Dysfunction

Changes in Urinary Patterns:

- Decreased urine output or frequency (oliguria)
- Increased urine output (polyuria), especially at night
- Foamy or bubbly urine
- Blood in the urine (hematuria)
- Difficulty or pain while urinating

Fluid Retention and Swelling (Edema):

- Swelling in the legs, ankles, feet, or face

- Sudden weight gain due to fluid retention
- Shortness of breath or difficulty breathing due to fluid buildup in the lungs (pulmonary edema)

Fatigue and Weakness:
- Generalized weakness and fatigue
- Difficulty concentrating or mental fog
- Feeling constantly tired or lethargic

Electrolyte Imbalance:
- Muscle cramps or twitching
- Nausea and vomiting
- Irregular heartbeat (arrhythmia)
- Tingling or numbness in the extremities

High Blood Pressure (Hypertension):
- Persistent high blood pressure readings
- Headaches
- Dizziness or lightheadedness

Bone and Joint Problems:
- Bone pain or tenderness
- Fractures or bone deformities
- Joint pain and stiffness

Skin Changes:
- Itchy skin (pruritus)
- Dry, flaky skin
- Pale skin or pallor
- Darkening or yellowing of the skin (jaundice) in severe cases

Other Symptoms:
- Loss of appetite
- Metallic taste in the mouth
- Difficulty sleeping
- Increased susceptibility to infections

Overview of Kidney Diseases

Kidney diseases, also known as renal diseases or nephropathies, encompass a wide range of conditions that affect the structure and function of the kidneys. The kidneys play a vital role in maintaining the body's overall health by filtering waste products and excess fluids from the blood, regulating electrolyte levels, and producing hormones that help control blood pressure and stimulate red blood cell production. When the kidneys become damaged or diseased, their ability to perform these essential functions may be impaired, leading to various health complications.

Types of Kidney Diseases:

Chronic Kidney Disease (CKD): CKD is a progressive condition characterized by the gradual loss of kidney function over time. It is typically diagnosed based on a persistent decrease in kidney function, measured by the glomerular filtration rate (GFR), or the presence of kidney damage for three months or more. CKD is categorized into five stages, with the final stage, known as end-stage renal disease (ESRD), requiring renal replacement therapy such as dialysis or kidney transplantation for survival.

Acute Kidney Injury (AKI): Also referred to as acute renal failure, AKI is a sudden and often reversible loss of kidney function that occurs over a short period, usually within a few hours or days. AKI can be caused by factors such as dehydration, severe infection, medication toxicity, or inadequate blood flow to the kidneys. Prompt diagnosis and treatment are essential to prevent further kidney damage and improve outcomes.

Polycystic Kidney Disease (PKD): PKD is a genetic disorder characterized by the growth of fluid-filled cysts in the kidneys, which can lead to kidney enlargement, high blood pressure, and kidney failure over time. There are two main types of PKD: autosomal dominant PKD (ADPKD), which is the most common form and usually develops in adulthood, and autosomal recessive PKD (ARPKD), which is rare and typically diagnosed in infancy or childhood.

Glomerulonephritis: Glomerulonephritis refers to inflammation of the glomeruli, the tiny filtering units in the kidneys responsible for removing waste and excess fluid from the blood. Glomerulonephritis can be acute or chronic and may result from infections, autoimmune diseases, or other underlying conditions. It can lead to proteinuria (protein in the urine), hematuria (blood in the urine), and decreased kidney function if left untreated.

Diabetic Nephropathy: Diabetic nephropathy is a common complication of both type 1 and type 2 diabetes and is a leading cause of CKD and ESRD worldwide. High blood sugar levels can damage the small blood vessels in the kidneys, impairing their ability to filter waste from the blood effectively. Diabetic nephropathy is characterized by proteinuria, high blood pressure, and progressive decline in kidney function.

Common Causes of Kidney Disease

Common causes of kidney disease can vary depending on the specific type of kidney disease. However, there are several overarching factors and conditions that can contribute to the development of kidney dysfunction.

Diabetes mellitus, both type 1 and type 2, is one of the leading causes of kidney disease. High blood sugar levels over time can damage the small blood vessels in the kidneys, impairing their ability to filter waste from the blood effectively. This condition, known as diabetic nephropathy, can lead to chronic kidney disease (CKD) and end-stage renal disease (ESRD) if left untreated.

Uncontrolled hypertension is another significant risk factor for kidney disease. High blood pressure can damage the blood vessels in the kidneys, leading to decreased kidney function over time. Conversely, kidney disease can also contribute to hypertension, creating a vicious cycle that further exacerbates kidney damage.

Glomerulonephritis refers to inflammation of the glomeruli, the tiny filtering units in the kidneys responsible for removing waste and excess fluid from the blood. This condition can be acute or chronic and may result from infections, autoimmune diseases, or other underlying conditions.

PKD is a genetic disorder characterized by the growth of fluid-filled cysts in the kidneys. These cysts can gradually enlarge and replace healthy kidney tissue, leading to kidney enlargement, high blood pressure, and eventually kidney failure. PKD can be inherited from one or both parents and typically manifests in adulthood.

Certain autoimmune diseases, such as lupus nephritis and vasculitis, can cause inflammation and damage to the kidneys. In these conditions, the body's immune system mistakenly attacks the kidneys, leading to decreased kidney function and potential complications.

Obstructions in the urinary tract, such as kidney stones, tumors, or enlarged prostate gland, can block the flow of urine and cause damage to the kidneys over time. Chronic obstruction can lead to hydronephrosis (swelling of the kidneys) and impaired kidney function.

Prolonged use of certain medications, such as nonsteroidal anti-inflammatory drugs (NSAIDs), certain antibiotics, and contrast agents used in medical imaging procedures, can cause kidney damage. Additionally, exposure to environmental toxins and heavy metals can also contribute to kidney dysfunction.

Other risk factors for kidney disease include aging, obesity, smoking, family history of kidney disease, and certain ethnic backgrounds (e.g., African American, Hispanic, Native American).

Dietary Guidelines

Instructions for Following a Dialysis Diet

Following a dialysis diet is crucial for managing kidney disease and optimizing treatment outcomes.

Monitor Fluid Intake: Individuals on dialysis need to closely monitor their fluid intake to prevent fluid overload, which can lead to complications such as high blood pressure, swelling, and shortness of breath. Your healthcare provider will provide guidance on the amount of fluid you should consume each day based on your individual needs.

Limit Sodium (Salt) Intake: Sodium can cause fluid retention and increase blood pressure, so it's important to limit sodium intake. Avoid adding salt to your meals and minimize consumption of processed and packaged foods, which are often high in sodium. Instead, opt for fresh fruits and vegetables, herbs, and spices to flavor your food.

Control Potassium Intake: Potassium is a mineral that can build up in the blood when kidney function is impaired. Too much potassium can lead to irregular heartbeats and other complications. Limit potassium-rich foods such as bananas, oranges, tomatoes, potatoes, and dairy products. Cooking certain high-potassium foods can help reduce their potassium content.

Monitor Phosphorus Intake: Phosphorus is a mineral that can accumulate in the blood when kidney function declines, leading to bone and heart problems. Limit phosphorus-rich foods such as dairy products, nuts, seeds, and processed foods. Your healthcare provider may also prescribe phosphate binders to help control phosphorus levels.

Watch Protein Intake: Dialysis patients need to consume enough protein to prevent malnutrition and support muscle health but may need to limit protein intake to reduce the build-up of waste products in the blood. Your healthcare provider or dietitian will recommend an appropriate amount of protein based on your individual needs.

Balance Carbohydrates: Carbohydrates are an important source of energy, but it's essential to choose complex carbohydrates such as whole grains, fruits, and vegetables over refined carbohydrates and sugary foods. Monitor carbohydrate intake to help control blood sugar levels if you have diabetes.

Follow Portion Control: Pay attention to portion sizes to avoid overeating and to help control calorie intake. Eating smaller, more frequent meals throughout the day may be helpful for managing appetite and blood sugar levels.

Take Vitamin and Mineral Supplements: Dialysis can lead to nutrient deficiencies, so your healthcare provider may recommend vitamin and mineral supplements, such as vitamin D, iron, and folic acid, to meet your nutritional needs.

Work with a Registered Dietitian: A registered dietitian specializing in renal nutrition can provide personalized guidance and meal planning tips to help you follow a dialysis diet tailored to your individual needs and preferences.

Stay Consistent and Keep Track: Consistency is key when following a dialysis diet. Keep track of your food and fluid intake, monitor your lab results, and communicate regularly with your healthcare team to make any necessary adjustments to your diet plan.

Strategies for Complying with Dietary Limitations

Complying with dietary limitations can be challenging, especially when following a specific diet such as a dialysis diet.

Understand the reasons behind your dietary limitations. Learn about how certain foods and nutrients can affect your health condition, and why it's important to adhere to dietary restrictions. Knowledge can empower you to make informed choices and stay motivated.

A registered dietitian specializing in renal nutrition can provide personalized guidance and support. They can help you understand your dietary limitations, create a customized meal plan, and offer practical tips for grocery shopping, meal preparation, and dining out.

Plan your meals and snacks ahead of time to ensure you have nutritious options available and to avoid impulsive food choices. Use your meal plan to create grocery lists and shop for ingredients accordingly. Meal planning can help you stay organized and committed to your dietary goals.

Explore new recipes that align with your dietary limitations. Look for kidney-friendly cookbooks, websites, and cooking videos for inspiration. Experiment with different ingredients, flavors, and cooking methods to keep your meals interesting and enjoyable.

Aim to include a variety of foods from different food groups in your diet to ensure you're getting a wide range of nutrients. Focus on incorporating lean proteins, whole grains, fruits, vegetables, and healthy fats into your meals. Strive for balance and moderation, rather than strict deprivation.

Adapt your favorite recipes to fit your dietary limitations. Substitute high-potassium or high-phosphorus ingredients with lower-phosphorus alternatives. Experiment with different herbs, spices, and seasoning blends to enhance flavor without relying on salt.

Pay attention to portion sizes to avoid overeating and to help control calorie intake. Use measuring cups, spoons, and food scales to accurately portion out your food. Eating smaller, more frequent meals throughout the day may help you feel satisfied without exceeding your dietary limits.

Drink water throughout the day to stay hydrated, especially if you're following fluid restrictions as part of your dietary limitations. Opt for water-rich foods such as fruits and vegetables to help satisfy thirst without exceeding fluid limits.

Focus on the foods you can eat rather than dwelling on those you need to avoid. Stay positive and celebrate your progress, no matter how small. Be flexible and open-minded, and don't be afraid to try new foods or adjust your meal plan as needed.

Surround yourself with supportive friends, family members, and healthcare professionals who understand your dietary limitations and can offer encouragement and assistance when needed. Joining support groups or online communities for individuals with similar dietary restrictions can also provide valuable resources and camaraderie.

30-Day Dialysis Diet Meal Plan

Weekly Meal Plan Summary

Monday:

Breakfast: Scrambled eggs with spinach and low-phosphorus toast

Snack: Greek yogurt with sliced strawberries

Lunch: Grilled chicken salad with mixed greens, bell peppers, and low-sodium vinaigrette

Snack: Carrot sticks with hummus

Dinner: Baked salmon with lemon, steamed green beans, and quinoa

Tuesday:

Breakfast: Oatmeal with sliced bananas and a sprinkle of cinnamon

Snack: Cottage cheese with pineapple chunks

Lunch: Turkey and avocado wrap with lettuce, tomato, and whole wheat tortilla

Snack: Apple slices with almond butter

Dinner: Stir-fried tofu with mixed vegetables and brown rice

Wednesday:

Breakfast: Whole grain cereal with low-fat milk and fresh blueberries

Snack: String cheese with whole grain crackers

Lunch: Lentil soup with a side of steamed asparagus

Snack: Trail mix with nuts, seeds, and dried fruit

Dinner: Grilled shrimp skewers with zucchini noodles and marinara sauce

Thursday:
Breakfast: Smoothie made with spinach, banana, low-potassium berries, and almond milk

Snack: Edamame (steamed soybeans)

Lunch: Quinoa salad with black beans, corn, cherry tomatoes, and lime vinaigrette

Snack: Rice cakes with avocado and tomato slices

Dinner: Baked chicken breast with roasted Brussels sprouts and sweet potato wedges

Friday:

Breakfast: Whole wheat toast with avocado and poached eggs

Snack: Cottage cheese with sliced peaches

Lunch: Tuna salad stuffed in a whole grain pita pocket with lettuce and cucumber

Snack: Air-popped popcorn

Dinner: Vegetable stir-fry with tofu or chicken and brown rice

Saturday:
Breakfast: Greek yogurt parfait with low-phosphorus granola and fresh berries

Snack: Celery sticks with peanut butter

Lunch: Whole grain pasta salad with cherry tomatoes, cucumbers, olives, and feta cheese

Snack: Mixed nuts

Dinner: Grilled steak with roasted cauliflower and quinoa pilaf

Sunday:

Breakfast: Veggie omelet with mushrooms, bell peppers, and onions

Snack: Pear slices with cheese

Lunch: Chicken Caesar salad with romaine lettuce, grilled chicken, Parmesan cheese, and low-sodium Caesar dressing

Snack: Sliced cucumbers with tzatziki sauce

Dinner: Baked fish with roasted vegetables and wild rice

Daily Meal Plans with Recipes and Portion Calculations

Monday:

Breakfast: Scrambled Eggs with Spinach and Whole Wheat Toast

- 2 large eggs
- 1 cup fresh spinach, chopped
- 1 teaspoon olive oil
- 1 slice whole wheat toast
- Calories: ~ 300 kcal
- Protein: ~ 20-25 grams

Snack: Greek Yogurt with Sliced Strawberries

- 1/2 cup plain Greek yogurt
- 1/2 cup sliced strawberries
- Calories: ~ 100 kcal
- Protein: ~ 10 grams

Lunch: Grilled Chicken Salad

- 3 oz grilled chicken breast
- 2 cups mixed greens
- 1/2 cup sliced bell peppers
- 2 tablespoons low-sodium vinaigrette
- Calories: ~ 300 kcal
- Protein: ~ 25-30 grams

Snack: Carrot Sticks with Hummus

- 1 medium carrot, sliced
- 2 tablespoons hummus
- Calories: ~ 100 kcal
- Protein: ~ 3-4 grams

Dinner: Baked Salmon with Lemon, Green Beans, and Quinoa

- 4 oz baked salmon with lemon
- 1 cup steamed green beans

- 1/2 cup cooked quinoa
- Calories: ~ 400 kcal
- Protein: ~ 25-30 grams

Tuesday:

Breakfast: Oatmeal with Sliced Bananas
- 1/2 cup rolled oats
- 1 cup water
- 1/2 medium banana, sliced
- Dash of cinnamon
- Calories: ~ 250 kcal
- Protein: ~ 5 grams

Snack: Cottage Cheese with Pineapple Chunks
- 1/2 cup low-fat cottage cheese
- 1/2 cup pineapple chunks (fresh or canned in juice)
- Calories: ~ 150 kcal

- Protein: ~ 15 grams

Lunch: Turkey and Avocado Wrap
- 3 oz sliced turkey breast
- 1/4 avocado, sliced
- 1 whole wheat tortilla
- Lettuce, tomato, and mustard (optional)
- Calories: ~ 300 kcal
- Protein: ~ 20-25 grams

Snack: Apple Slices with Almond Butter
- 1 small apple, sliced
- 2 tablespoons almond butter
- Calories: ~ 200 kcal
- Protein: ~ 5-7 grams

Dinner: Stir-Fried Tofu with Mixed Vegetables and Brown Rice
- 4 oz tofu, cubed

- 1 cup mixed vegetables (such as bell peppers, broccoli, and snap peas)
- 1/2 cup cooked brown rice
- Low-sodium soy sauce for seasoning
- Calories: ~ 400 kcal
- Protein: ~ 15-20 grams

Recipes

Meal Ideas for Breakfast

1. Scrambled Eggs with Spinach and Whole Wheat Toast:
- Scramble 2 large eggs with chopped fresh spinach in 1 teaspoon of olive oil. Serve with a slice of whole wheat toast.
- This meal provides protein from eggs and spinach, as well as fiber and carbohydrates from whole wheat toast.

2. Oatmeal with Sliced Bananas and Cinnamon:
- Cook 1/2 cup of rolled oats with 1 cup of water. Top with sliced bananas and a dash of cinnamon.

- Oatmeal is a good source of fiber and complex carbohydrates, while bananas add natural sweetness and potassium.

3. Greek Yogurt Parfait with Low-Phosphorus Granola and Berries:
- Layer 1/2 cup of plain Greek yogurt with low-phosphorus granola and fresh berries (such as strawberries, blueberries, or raspberries).
- Greek yogurt provides protein, while granola and berries add crunch and flavor without excess phosphorus.

4. Whole Grain Toast with Avocado and Poached Eggs:
- Toast a slice of whole grain bread and top with mashed avocado and a poached egg.

- Avocado adds healthy fats, while poached eggs provide protein and nutrients.

5. Smoothie with Spinach, Banana, and Low-Potassium Berries:
- Blend together a handful of spinach, 1/2 banana, and a small portion of low-potassium berries (such as raspberries or strawberries) with water or almond milk.
- Smoothies are a convenient way to pack in nutrients, and spinach adds iron and vitamins.

6. Low-Potassium Pancakes with Fresh Fruit Topping:
- Make pancakes using a low-potassium pancake mix or recipe, and top with fresh fruit such as sliced peaches, kiwi, or melon.

- Low-potassium pancakes can be made using alternatives to traditional ingredients like bananas or yogurt.

7. Cottage Cheese with Sliced Pineapple:
- Enjoy 1/2 cup of low-fat cottage cheese with sliced pineapple.
- Cottage cheese is a good source of protein, while pineapple adds natural sweetness and vitamin C.

8. Vegetable Omelet with Whole Wheat Toast:
- Make an omelet with chopped vegetables such as bell peppers, onions, and mushrooms. Serve with a slice of whole wheat toast.

- Vegetables add fiber and nutrients, while eggs provide protein for a satisfying breakfast.

Lunch Recipes

1. Grilled Chicken Salad:

Ingredients:

- 3 oz grilled chicken breast, sliced
- 2 cups mixed greens
- 1/2 cup sliced bell peppers
- 1/4 cup sliced cucumber
- 2 tablespoons low-sodium vinaigrette

Instructions:

1. Grill chicken breast until cooked through, then slice.
2. In a large bowl, combine mixed greens, sliced bell peppers, and sliced cucumber.

3. Top the salad with sliced grilled chicken breast.

4. Drizzle with low-sodium vinaigrette and toss to coat. Serve immediately.

2. Turkey and Avocado Wrap:

Ingredients:

- 3 oz sliced turkey breast
- 1/4 avocado, sliced
- 1 whole wheat tortilla
-Lettuce, tomato, and mustard (optional)

Instructions:

1. Lay the whole wheat tortilla flat.

2. Layer sliced turkey breast, avocado slices, lettuce, tomato, and mustard (if desired) on the tortilla.

3. Roll up the tortilla tightly, then slice in half diagonally. Serve immediately.

Quinoa Salad with Black Beans and Corn:

Ingredients:
- 1/2 cup cooked quinoa
- 1/4 cup black beans, drained and rinsed
- 1/4 cup corn kernels (fresh, frozen, or canned)
- 2 tablespoons diced red onion
- 2 tablespoons chopped fresh cilantro
- 1 tablespoon lime juice
- Salt and pepper to taste

Instructions:
1. In a bowl, combine cooked quinoa, black beans, corn kernels, diced red onion, and chopped fresh cilantro.
2. Drizzle with lime juice and season with salt and pepper to taste. Toss to combine.

3. Serve the quinoa salad chilled or at room temperature.

Tuna Salad Stuffed Pita Pocket:
Ingredients:
- 1 whole wheat pita pocket
- 1/2 cup canned tuna, drained
- 1 tablespoon plain Greek yogurt
- 1/4 cup diced cucumber
- 1/4 cup diced tomato
- 1 tablespoon chopped fresh parsley
- Salt and pepper to taste

Instructions:
1. In a bowl, mix together canned tuna, plain Greek yogurt, diced cucumber, diced tomato, chopped fresh parsley, salt, and pepper.

2. Cut the whole wheat pita pocket in half to form two pockets.

3. Stuff each pita pocket with the tuna salad mixture. Serve immediately.

Lentil Soup:
Ingredients:
- 1/2 cup dried lentils, rinsed and drained
- 2 cups low-sodium vegetable broth
- 1/2 cup diced carrots
- 1/2 cup diced celery
- 1/4 cup diced onion
- 1 clove garlic, minced
- 1 bay leaf
- Salt and pepper to taste

Instructions:

1. In a pot, combine dried lentils, low-sodium vegetable broth, diced carrots, diced celery, diced onion, minced garlic, and bay leaf.

2. Bring the mixture to a boil, then reduce heat and simmer for 20-25 minutes, or until lentils are tender.

3. Season with salt and pepper to taste. Remove the bay leaf before serving.

10 Dialysis Patient Breakfast Ideas
Scrambled Eggs with Spinach and Whole Wheat Toast:
- Scrambled eggs cooked with chopped spinach, served with a slice of whole wheat toast.

Oatmeal with Sliced Bananas and Cinnamon:

- Cooked oatmeal topped with sliced bananas and a sprinkle of cinnamon.

Greek Yogurt Parfait with Low-Phosphorus Granola and Berries:

- Layered Greek yogurt, low-phosphorus granola, and fresh berries (such as strawberries or blueberries).

Whole Grain Toast with Avocado and Poached Eggs:

- Whole grain toast topped with mashed avocado and poached eggs.

Smoothie with Spinach, Banana, and Low-Potassium Berries:
- Blend together spinach, banana, low-potassium berries (such as raspberries or strawberries), and water or almond milk.

Low-Potassium Pancakes with Fresh Fruit Topping:
- Pancakes made with a low-potassium mix, topped with fresh fruit (such as sliced peaches or berries).

Cottage Cheese with Sliced Pineapple:
- Low-fat cottage cheese served with sliced pineapple.

Vegetable Omelet with Whole Wheat Toast:

- Omelet made with chopped vegetables (such as bell peppers, onions, and mushrooms) served with whole wheat toast.

Whole Grain Cereal with Low-Fat Milk and Fresh Berries:
- Whole grain cereal served with low-fat milk and fresh berries (such as blueberries or raspberries).

Low-Potassium Breakfast Burrito:
- Whole wheat tortilla filled with scrambled eggs, diced vegetables, and salsa.

Dinner Recipes

Baked Salmon with Lemon and Herbs:
Ingredients:
- 4 oz salmon fillet
- 1 tablespoon olive oil

- 1 tablespoon fresh lemon juice
- 1 teaspoon chopped fresh dill
- Salt and pepper to taste

Instructions:

1. Preheat the oven to 375°F (190°C).

2. Place the salmon fillet on a baking sheet lined with parchment paper.

3. Drizzle olive oil and lemon juice over the salmon.

4. Sprinkle chopped fresh dill, salt, and pepper on top.

5. Bake for 15-20 minutes, or until the salmon is cooked through and flakes easily with a fork.

Grilled Chicken with Roasted Vegetables:

Ingredients:

- 4 oz chicken breast
- 1 cup mixed vegetables (such as bell peppers, zucchini, and onions), diced
- 1 tablespoon olive oil
- 1 teaspoon Italian seasoning
- Salt and pepper to taste

Instructions:

1. Preheat the grill or grill pan over medium heat.

2. Season the chicken breast with Italian seasoning, salt, and pepper.

3. Grill the chicken breast for 6-8 minutes on each side, or until cooked through.

4. Meanwhile, toss the diced vegetables with olive oil, salt, and pepper.

5. Spread the vegetables on a baking sheet and roast in the oven at 400°F (200°C) for 20-25 minutes, or until tender.

6. Serve the grilled chicken with roasted vegetables on the side.

Vegetable Stir-Fry with Tofu:
Ingredients:
- 4 oz firm tofu, cubed
- 2 cups mixed vegetables (such as broccoli, carrots, and snap peas), sliced
- 2 tablespoons low-sodium soy sauce
- 1 tablespoon sesame oil
- 1 teaspoon minced garlic

- Cooked brown rice for serving

Instructions:

1. Heat sesame oil in a large skillet or wok over medium heat.

2. Add minced garlic and cubed tofu to the skillet, and cook until tofu is lightly browned.

3. Add mixed vegetables to the skillet and stir-fry for 5-7 minutes, or until vegetables are tender-crisp.

4. Stir in low-sodium soy sauce and cook for an additional 1-2 minutes.

5. Serve the vegetable stir-fry with cooked brown rice.

Turkey Meatballs with Marinara Sauce:

Ingredients:

- 4 oz ground turkey

-1/4 cup breadcrumbs (preferably whole wheat)

-1 tablespoon grated Parmesan cheese

-1/2 teaspoon Italian seasoning

- Salt and pepper to taste

- 1 cup low-sodium marinara sauce

Instructions:

1. Preheat the oven to 375°F (190°C).

2. In a bowl, combine ground turkey, breadcrumbs, Parmesan cheese, Italian seasoning, salt, and pepper.

3. Shape the mixture into meatballs and place them on a baking sheet lined with parchment paper.

4. Bake for 20-25 minutes, or until the meatballs are cooked through.

5. Heat the marinara sauce in a saucepan over medium heat.

6. Serve the turkey meatballs with marinara sauce over cooked whole wheat pasta or spaghetti squash.

Quinoa Salad with Black Beans and Corn:

Ingredients:
- 1/2 cup cooked quinoa

- 1/4 cup black beans, drained and rinsed
- 1/4 cup corn kernels (fresh, frozen, or canned)
- 2 tablespoons diced red onion
- 2 tablespoons chopped fresh cilantro
- 1 tablespoon lime juice
- Salt and pepper to taste

Instructions:

1. In a bowl, combine cooked quinoa, black beans, corn kernels, diced red onion, and chopped fresh cilantro.

2. Drizzle with lime juice and season with salt and pepper to taste. Toss to combine.

3. Serve the quinoa salad chilled or at room temperature.

10 Lunch Ideas for Dialysis Patients

1. Grilled Chicken Salad:
- Grilled chicken breast slices served over mixed greens with cherry tomatoes, cucumbers, and a light vinaigrette dressing.

2. Tuna Salad Lettuce Wraps:
- Tuna salad made with canned tuna, Greek yogurt, diced celery, and spices, wrapped in lettuce leaves for a low-carb, protein-rich meal.

3. Vegetable and Lentil Soup:
- Homemade soup made with low-sodium vegetable broth, lentils, carrots, celery, onions, and spinach, seasoned with herbs and spices.

4. Quinoa and Black Bean Bowl:

- Cooked quinoa mixed with black beans, diced bell peppers, corn kernels, and avocado slices, drizzled with lime juice and topped with cilantro.

5. Grilled Salmon with Steamed Vegetables:
- Grilled salmon fillet served with a side of steamed broccoli, cauliflower, and carrots, seasoned with herbs and lemon.

6. Turkey and Hummus Wrap:
- Whole wheat wrap filled with sliced turkey breast, hummus, lettuce, tomato, and cucumber, rolled up for a satisfying and protein-packed meal.

7. Greek Yogurt and Fruit Parfait:
- Layered Greek yogurt with low-sugar granola, fresh berries, and a drizzle of honey

or maple syrup for a nutritious and delicious treat.

8. Egg Salad Sandwich:
- Egg salad made with hard-boiled eggs, Greek yogurt, mustard, and diced celery, served on whole grain bread with lettuce and tomato.

9. Caprese Salad with Balsamic Glaze:
- Sliced tomatoes, fresh mozzarella cheese, and basil leaves drizzled with balsamic glaze, served as a light and refreshing salad.

10. Vegetable Stir-Fry with Tofu:
- Stir-fried tofu with mixed vegetables (such as bell peppers, broccoli, and snap peas) in a light soy sauce, served over brown rice or quinoa for a satisfying and nutritious meal.

Snack Recipes

1. Apple and Almond Butter Slices:

Ingredients:

- 1 medium apple, sliced
- 2 tablespoons almond butter

Instructions:

1. Spread almond butter on apple slices.

2. Enjoy as a satisfying and nutritious snack.

2. Carrot Sticks with Hummus:

Ingredients:

- 2 medium carrots, peeled and cut into sticks
- 1/4 cup hummus

Instructions:

1. Serve carrot sticks with hummus for a crunchy and protein-rich snack.

3. Greek Yogurt with Berries and Nuts:
Ingredients:
- 1/2 cup plain Greek yogurt
- 1/4 cup mixed berries (such as strawberries, blueberries, or raspberries)
- 1 tablespoon chopped nuts (such as almonds or walnuts)

Instructions:
1. Top Greek yogurt with mixed berries and chopped nuts for a balanced and satisfying snack.

4. Cottage Cheese with Pineapple Chunks:

Ingredients:

- 1/2 cup low-fat cottage cheese

- 1/2 cup pineapple chunks (fresh or canned in juice)

Instructions:

1. Serve low-fat cottage cheese with pineapple chunks for a protein-packed and refreshing snack.

5. Homemade Trail Mix:

Ingredients:

- 1/4 cup mixed nuts (such as almonds, walnuts, and cashews)

- 1/4 cup dried fruit (such as raisins, cranberries, or apricots)

- 1/4 cup whole grain cereal or pretzel sticks

Instructions:

1. Mix together nuts, dried fruit, and whole grain cereal or pretzel sticks to create a customized trail mix.

2. Portion into small snack bags for a convenient grab-and-go option.

10 Dinner Ideas for Dialysis Patients

1. Grilled Chicken Breast with Roasted Vegetables:- Grilled chicken breast seasoned with herbs and spices, served with roasted vegetables such as broccoli, carrots, and bell peppers.

2. Baked Salmon with Lemon and Dill:- Baked salmon fillet seasoned with lemon

juice, dill, and garlic, served with a side of steamed green beans or asparagus.

3. Turkey Meatballs with Marinara Sauce:- Turkey meatballs made with lean ground turkey, breadcrumbs, and Italian seasoning, served with low-sodium marinara sauce over whole wheat pasta or spaghetti squash.

4. Vegetable Stir-Fry with Tofu:- Stir-fried tofu with mixed vegetables (such as bell peppers, snap peas, and mushrooms) in a light soy sauce, served over brown rice or quinoa.

5. Lentil Soup with Whole Grain Bread:- Homemade lentil soup made with low-sodium vegetable broth, lentils, carrots,

celery, onions, and spices, served with a slice of whole grain bread.

6. Grilled Shrimp Skewers with Quinoa Salad:- Grilled shrimp skewers seasoned with lemon and garlic, served with a quinoa salad made with black beans, corn, tomatoes, and cilantro.

7. Chicken and Vegetable Curry:- Chicken and vegetable curry made with boneless, skinless chicken breast, curry paste, coconut milk, and mixed vegetables, served over brown rice.

8. Baked Cod with Herbed Quinoa Pilaf:- Baked cod fillet seasoned with fresh herbs and lemon zest, served with a quinoa pilaf made with diced vegetables and herbs.

9. Vegetarian Chili with Cornbread Muffins:- Vegetarian chili made with kidney beans, black beans, diced tomatoes, bell peppers, onions, and spices, served with whole grain cornbread muffins.

10. Greek Salad with Grilled Lamb Chops:- Greek salad made with mixed greens, cucumber, tomato, red onion, olives, and feta cheese, served with grilled lamb chops seasoned with oregano and garlic.

Easy and Nutritious Snack Ideas

1. Greek Yogurt with Honey and Almonds:- Serve plain Greek yogurt drizzled with honey and sprinkled with sliced almonds for a protein-rich and satisfying snack.

2. Fruit and Cheese Plate:- Pair sliced apples, pears, or grapes with low-sodium cheese cubes or slices for a balanced snack that combines carbohydrates, protein, and fiber.

3. Vegetable Sticks with Hummus:- Dip carrot sticks, cucumber slices, bell pepper strips, and cherry tomatoes in hummus for a crunchy and fiber-filled snack.

4. Hard-Boiled Eggs:- Enjoy hard-boiled eggs as a portable and protein-packed snack option. Sprinkle with a pinch of salt and pepper for extra flavor.

5. Trail Mix with Nuts and Dried Fruit:- Mix together unsalted nuts (such as almonds, walnuts, and cashews) with dried fruit (such

as raisins, apricots, and cranberries) for a nutrient-dense snack on the go.

6. Rice Cake with Peanut Butter and Banana Slices:- Spread natural peanut butter on a rice cake and top with sliced bananas for a satisfying and energy-boosting snack.

7. Cottage Cheese with Pineapple Chunks:- Enjoy a serving of low-fat cottage cheese with canned pineapple chunks (packed in juice) for a creamy and tropical-flavored snack.

8. Whole Grain Crackers with Tuna Salad:- Top whole grain crackers with homemade tuna salad made with canned tuna, Greek yogurt, diced celery, and mustard for a protein-rich snack option.

9. Edamame Pods:- Steam edamame pods and sprinkle with sea salt for a flavorful and nutritious snack that's rich in plant-based protein and fiber.

10. Smoothie with Spinach and Berries:- Blend together fresh spinach, frozen berries, Greek yogurt, and a splash of almond milk for a refreshing and nutrient-packed smoothie.

Kidney Health and Dialysis

Overview of Dialysis Treatment

Dialysis treatment is a life-saving procedure used to manage kidney failure, also known as end-stage renal disease (ESRD), when the kidneys are no longer able to function effectively. Dialysis helps to remove waste products, excess fluid, and toxins from the blood, restoring the body's balance of electrolytes and fluids.

Hemodialysis

In hemodialysis, blood is removed from the body and circulated through a dialysis machine, also called an artificial kidney. Within the machine, the blood passes through a special filter called a dialyzer, which acts as an artificial kidney to remove waste products and excess fluids. The cleaned blood is then returned to the body. Hemodialysis is typically performed three times per week in a dialysis center or at home under the supervision of healthcare professionals.

Peritoneal Dialysis

Peritoneal dialysis involves using the lining of the abdomen, called the peritoneum, as a natural filter. A sterile solution called dialysate is infused into the abdomen through a catheter. The dialysate absorbs waste products and excess fluids from the blood vessels lining the peritoneum. After a period of dwell time, the used dialysate is drained from the abdomen, carrying waste products and excess fluids out of the body. Peritoneal dialysis can be performed at home, allowing for more flexibility in treatment schedules.

Dialysis treatment aims to:
- Remove waste products, excess fluids, and toxins from the blood.
- Maintain the balance of electrolytes such as sodium, potassium, and calcium in the body.
- Control blood pressure and fluid balance.
- Help manage symptoms and complications associated with kidney failure.

Function of Healthy Kidneys
Filtration of Waste Products:
The kidneys filter waste products, toxins, and excess substances (such as sodium,

potassium, and urea) from the bloodstream. These waste products are then excreted from the body in the form of urine.

Regulation of Fluid Balance

The kidneys help regulate the body's fluid balance by adjusting the volume and concentration of urine produced. This helps maintain proper hydration and blood pressure levels.

Control of Electrolyte Levels

Kidneys regulate the levels of electrolytes, such as sodium, potassium, calcium, and phosphate, in the bloodstream. Proper electrolyte balance is essential for normal nerve and muscle function, as well as maintaining proper pH levels in the body.

Production of Hormones

The kidneys produce several hormones that play important roles in regulating various bodily functions, including:

Renin: Regulates blood pressure by controlling the constriction and dilation of blood vessels.

Erythropoietin (EPO): Stimulates the production of red blood cells in the bone marrow.

Calcitriol (active form of vitamin D): Helps regulate calcium levels and maintain bone health.

Acid-Base Balance

Kidneys help regulate the body's acid-base balance by excreting hydrogen ions and reabsorbing bicarbonate ions, which helps maintain the pH balance of bodily fluids.

Blood Pressure Regulation

The kidneys help regulate blood pressure by controlling the volume of blood circulating in the body and by producing hormones that influence blood vessel constriction and dilation.

Detoxification

In addition to filtering waste products from the blood, the kidneys also help detoxify the body by eliminating drugs, medications, and other harmful substances.

Dietary Basics for Patients Receiving Dialysis

Value of a Balanced Diet

A balanced diet provides numerous benefits for overall health and well-being.

A balanced diet ensures that your body receives all the essential nutrients it needs in the right proportions. This includes carbohydrates, proteins, fats, vitamins, minerals, and water. Each nutrient plays a specific role in supporting various bodily functions, from energy production to immune function and tissue repair.

Consuming a balanced diet provides your body with the necessary fuel to maintain energy levels throughout the day.

Carbohydrates are the body's primary source of energy, while fats and proteins also contribute to energy production. By consuming a variety of nutrient-rich foods, you can sustain consistent energy levels and avoid energy crashes.

A balanced diet can help you achieve and maintain a healthy weight. By incorporating a variety of nutrient-dense foods such as fruits, vegetables, lean proteins, and whole grains, you can feel satisfied and maintain a healthy calorie balance. Additionally, a balanced diet can support metabolic health and reduce the risk of obesity-related diseases.

Consuming a variety of fiber-rich foods such as fruits, vegetables, whole grains, and legumes can promote digestive health by preventing constipation, supporting regular bowel movements, and maintaining a healthy gut microbiome. Adequate fiber intake also helps reduce the risk of gastrointestinal disorders such as diverticulosis and hemorrhoids.

A balanced diet rich in vitamins, minerals, and antioxidants supports a strong immune system, helping your body defend against infections and illnesses. Nutrients such as vitamin C, vitamin D, zinc, and selenium play crucial roles in immune function and can be obtained from a variety of fruits, vegetables, nuts, seeds, and lean meats.

Following a balanced diet can help reduce the risk of chronic diseases such as heart disease, type 2 diabetes, hypertension, and certain cancers. By emphasizing whole foods and limiting processed foods high in unhealthy fats, sugars, and sodium, you can promote heart health, maintain healthy blood sugar levels, and support overall longevity.

Nutrient-rich foods can positively impact mental health and cognitive function. Essential nutrients such as omega-3 fatty acids, vitamins B6 and B12, and folate play roles in neurotransmitter synthesis and brain function. Consuming a balanced diet that includes sources of these nutrients may help reduce the risk of depression, anxiety, and cognitive decline.

Foods to Restrict and Steer Clear of

High-Sodium Foods

Excessive sodium intake can contribute to high blood pressure and increase the risk of heart disease and stroke. Foods high in sodium include processed meats (such as bacon, sausage, and deli meats), canned soups and broths, salty snacks (like chips and pretzels), processed and packaged foods, and fast food. It's important to read food labels and choose low-sodium or sodium-free options whenever possible.

High-Sugar Foods and Beverages

Consuming too much sugar can contribute to weight gain, obesity, type 2 diabetes, and dental cavities. Foods high in added sugars include sugary beverages (such as soda, fruit juice, and sweetened tea or coffee), candy, baked goods (like cakes, cookies, and pastries), sugary cereals, and flavored yogurt. Opt for naturally sweet foods like fresh fruit or choose products with no added sugars.

Trans Fats and Saturated Fats

Trans fats and saturated fats can raise levels of LDL cholesterol (often referred to as "bad" cholesterol) and increase the risk of heart disease. Foods high in trans fats include fried foods, commercial baked goods (such as cookies, pastries, and doughnuts), margarine, and some processed snacks. Saturated fats are found in high-fat dairy products, fatty cuts of meat, butter, and coconut oil. Instead, choose healthier fats like monounsaturated and polyunsaturated fats found in nuts, seeds, avocados, and olive oil.

High-Phosphorus Foods

Individuals with kidney disease, particularly those on dialysis, may need to restrict their intake of phosphorus-rich foods to avoid complications such as bone and heart problems. High-phosphorus foods include dairy products, nuts, seeds, whole grains, chocolate, processed meats, and carbonated beverages. It's important for individuals with kidney disease to work closely with a healthcare provider or dietitian to manage phosphorus levels in their diet.

High-Potassium Foods

For individuals with kidney disease, especially those with advanced kidney failure, high-potassium foods can cause dangerous electrolyte imbalances. High-potassium foods include bananas, oranges, potatoes (especially sweet potatoes), tomatoes, spinach, avocados, and dried fruits. People with kidney disease may need to limit their intake of these foods and choose lower-potassium alternatives.

Alcohol

Excessive alcohol consumption can have negative effects on overall health, including liver damage, heart problems, and increased risk of certain cancers. It can also interact with medications and exacerbate certain health conditions. It's best to consume alcohol in moderation or avoid it altogether, particularly for individuals with liver disease, heart disease, or a history of substance abuse.

Tips and Strategies for Meal Planning

Strategies for Successful Meal Planning

Successful meal planning involves careful consideration of dietary needs, preferences, and lifestyle factors.

Determine your dietary goals and priorities, such as eating more vegetables, reducing sodium intake, or incorporating more home-cooked meals. Setting achievable goals will guide your meal planning efforts and keep you motivated.

Understand your nutritional requirements based on factors such as age, gender, activity level, and any underlying health conditions.

Consider consulting with a healthcare provider or registered dietitian to assess your specific nutritional needs.

Plan your meals for the upcoming week, considering breakfast, lunch, dinner, and snacks. Start by selecting a variety of recipes and meals that align with your dietary goals and nutritional needs. Aim for balance and diversity by including a mix of protein sources, whole grains, fruits, vegetables, and healthy fats.

Once you have your meal plan in place, create a shopping list based on the ingredients needed for your recipes. Organize your list by food categories (e.g., produce, proteins, pantry items) to streamline your grocery shopping trip and avoid forgetting essential ingredients.

Dedicate time each week to prepping ingredients in advance, such as washing and chopping vegetables, cooking grains, and marinating proteins. Prepping ingredients ahead of time can save time during busy weekdays and make meal preparation more efficient.

Consider batch cooking large quantities of staple ingredients, such as grains, proteins, and sauces, to use throughout the week. Cook once and enjoy multiple meals by incorporating these pre-cooked components into different recipes.

Take advantage of time-saving kitchen tools and appliances, such as a slow cooker, pressure cooker, or food processor, to streamline meal preparation. These tools can help you cook meals more quickly and with less hands-on effort.

Invest in a set of meal prep containers to portion out and store pre-cooked meals and ingredients. Having meals ready to grab and go can help you stick to your meal plan, even on busy days.

Be flexible and adaptable with your meal plan to accommodate changes in schedule, unexpected events, or last-minute cravings. Consider keeping a variety of versatile ingredients on hand that can be used interchangeably in different recipes.

Keep track of your meals and their impact on your energy levels, hunger, and satisfaction. Reflect on what worked well and what could be improved, and make adjustments to your meal plan accordingly for future weeks.

Buying Advice for Dialysis

When it comes to purchasing items related to dialysis, whether for home dialysis treatment or to support someone undergoing dialysis, there are several important considerations to keep in mind.

1. Consult with Healthcare Providers: Before making any purchases related to dialysis, it's crucial to consult with healthcare providers, including nephrologists, dialysis nurses, and dietitians. They can provide guidance on

specific equipment, supplies, and dietary needs based on individual medical conditions and treatment plans.

2. Research Home Dialysis Options: If considering home dialysis, such as peritoneal dialysis or home hemodialysis, research the available options thoroughly. Consider factors such as equipment requirements, training and support provided by dialysis clinics or equipment suppliers, and insurance coverage for home dialysis treatments.

3. Compare Equipment and Supplies: When purchasing dialysis equipment and supplies, such as dialysis machines, peritoneal dialysis catheters, dialysate solutions, and dialysis accessories, compare products from

different manufacturers. Consider factors such as quality, reliability, ease of use, compatibility with existing equipment, and cost.

4. Evaluate Safety and Sterility: Ensure that any equipment or supplies used for dialysis treatment meet safety and sterility standards. Look for products that are FDA-approved, CE-marked (for European countries), or compliant with other relevant regulatory standards. Follow proper procedures for cleaning and disinfecting equipment to prevent infections and complications.

5. Consider Convenience and Accessibility: Choose products and supplies that offer convenience and accessibility for the

individual undergoing dialysis. This may include portable or compact dialysis equipment for travel or on-the-go use, easy-to-handle supplies, and storage solutions to keep supplies organized and accessible.

6. Check Insurance Coverage: Before purchasing dialysis-related equipment, supplies, or medications, check with insurance providers to understand coverage and reimbursement policies. Some insurance plans may cover certain dialysis-related expenses, including equipment, supplies, medications, and home healthcare services.

7. Seek Financial Assistance: For individuals facing financial challenges related to dialysis

treatment, inquire about financial assistance programs offered by government agencies, nonprofit organizations, dialysis clinics, and pharmaceutical companies. These programs may provide financial support, discounts, or subsidies for dialysis-related expenses.

8. Read Reviews and Seek Recommendations: Before making a purchase, read reviews and seek recommendations from healthcare professionals, patient support groups, online forums, and community resources. Hearing from others who have experience with specific products or suppliers can provide valuable insights and help inform purchasing decisions.

9. Plan for Long-Term Needs: Consider the long-term needs and sustainability of dialysis treatment when purchasing equipment and supplies. Choose products and suppliers that offer reliable support, maintenance, and replacement services to ensure continuous access to dialysis treatment over time.

10. Prioritize Patient Comfort and Well-Being: Above all, prioritize patient comfort, safety, and well-being when selecting dialysis equipment, supplies, and support services. Choose products and solutions that enhance quality of life, promote independence, and support overall health and wellness for individuals undergoing dialysis.

Friendly Foods

"Kidney-friendly" or "dialysis-friendly" foods are those that are low in sodium, phosphorus, and potassium, making them suitable for individuals with kidney disease, especially those undergoing dialysis.

1. Fruits:

- Apples (with skin removed)
- Berries (e.g., strawberries, blueberries, raspberries)
- Pineapple
- Grapes
-Watermelon (in moderation)
- Cranberries (in limited amounts)

2. Vegetables:
 - Leafy greens (e.g., spinach, kale, lettuce)
- Bell peppers
- Cabbage

- Cauliflower
- Broccoli
- Green beans
- Zucchini
- Cucumber

3. Proteins:
- Skinless chicken or turkey
- Fish (e.g., salmon, cod, tilapia)
- Eggs (in moderation)
- Tofu
- Lean cuts of beef or pork (in moderation)

4. Grains and Starches:
- White bread (in moderation)
- White rice (in moderation)
- Pasta (in moderation)
- Rice cakes

- Corn or rice-based cereals (low in potassium)
- Oatmeal (in moderation)

5. Dairy and Dairy Alternatives:
- Low-fat or fat-free milk
- Low-fat or fat-free yogurt
- Low-fat or fat-free cheese (in moderation)
- Dairy alternatives (e.g., almond milk, rice milk, soy milk)

6. Snacks:
- Air-popped popcorn (in moderation)
- Rice cakes with nut butter
- Homemade trail mix with unsalted nuts and dried fruits (in moderation)
- Low-sodium crackers or pretzels
- Fresh fruit slices with a small amount of nut butter

7. Beverages:

- Water (best choice)

- Herbal teas (unsweetened)

- Coffee (in moderation)

- Fruit juices (diluted and in limited amounts)

- Lemonade or limeade (made with sugar substitute)

Special Considerations and Tips

Managing Nutritional Difficulties

Managing nutritional difficulties, especially for individuals with health conditions such as kidney disease or undergoing dialysis, requires careful planning and consideration of dietary restrictions.

1. Consult with Healthcare Providers: Seek guidance from healthcare professionals, including nephrologists, dietitians, and nurses, who specialize in managing specific health conditions such as kidney disease or diabetes. They can provide personalized recommendations based on individual health status, medical history, and dietary needs.

2. Follow a Customized Meal Plan: Work with a registered dietitian to develop a customized meal plan tailored to your specific nutritional needs and dietary restrictions. A well-balanced meal plan will take into account factors such as protein,

sodium, potassium, phosphorus, and fluid intake, while ensuring adequate nutrition and energy levels.

3. Monitor Nutrient Intake: Keep track of your daily nutrient intake, including protein, sodium, potassium, phosphorus, and fluid intake. Use tools such as food journals or mobile apps to record food choices and portion sizes, and monitor changes in nutritional parameters over time.

4. Limit Sodium Intake: Reduce sodium intake by avoiding high-sodium processed foods, canned soups, packaged snacks, and salty condiments. Instead, choose fresh or minimally processed foods, use herbs and spices to flavor dishes, and opt for

low-sodium or sodium-free alternatives when available.

5. Manage Potassium and Phosphorus: Limit potassium-rich foods such as bananas, oranges, tomatoes, potatoes, and dairy products if you have elevated potassium levels. Similarly, restrict phosphorus-rich foods like dairy products, nuts, seeds, and processed meats to manage phosphorus levels effectively.

6. Control Fluid Intake: Monitor fluid intake to avoid fluid overload, especially for individuals with kidney disease or heart failure. Limit consumption of high-fluid foods such as soups, stews, and juicy fruits, and follow fluid restrictions prescribed by healthcare providers.

7. Optimize Protein Intake: Consume high-quality protein sources such as lean meats, poultry, fish, eggs, tofu, and low-fat dairy products to meet protein needs while minimizing phosphorus intake. Consider working with a dietitian to determine the appropriate amount of protein for your individual requirements.

8. Manage Blood Sugar Levels: If you have diabetes or insulin resistance, monitor blood sugar levels closely and follow a diabetic-friendly meal plan that emphasizes whole grains, lean proteins, non-starchy vegetables, and healthy fats. Avoid sugary foods and beverages that can spike blood sugar levels.

9. Address Nutritional Deficiencies: Address any nutritional deficiencies through dietary modifications, supplementation, or medications as recommended by healthcare providers. Common deficiencies in individuals with kidney disease may include vitamin D, iron, and B vitamins.

10. Stay Educated and Informed: Stay informed about nutrition guidelines, dietary recommendations, and new research developments related to managing specific health conditions. Attend educational sessions, workshops, or support groups to learn more about nutrition and dietary strategies for managing nutritional difficulties effectively.

Advice for Dialysis Patients When Dining Out

Dining out can present challenges for individuals undergoing dialysis, as it may be difficult to find kidney-friendly options on restaurant menus. However, with some careful planning and preparation, dialysis patients can still enjoy dining out while managing their dietary restrictions effectively.

1. Choose Restaurants Wisely: Select restaurants that offer a variety of menu options and are willing to accommodate special dietary requests. Look for restaurants that prioritize fresh, whole ingredients and allow for customization of dishes.

2. Plan Ahead: Before dining out, research the restaurant's menu online or call ahead to inquire about kidney-friendly options and modifications. Look for dishes that are lower in sodium, potassium, and phosphorus, and ask if substitutions or adjustments can be made to meet your dietary needs.

3. Ask Questions: Don't hesitate to ask your server or the restaurant staff about the ingredients, cooking methods, and portion sizes of menu items. Request modifications such as omitting high-sodium sauces, dressings, or condiments, and opting for grilled or steamed preparations instead of fried or breaded dishes.

4. Customize Your Order: Be proactive in customizing your order to make it more kidney-friendly. Request sauces, dressings, and toppings on the side so you can control the amount added to your meal. Ask for substitutions such as steamed vegetables or a side salad instead of high-potassium side dishes like French fries or mashed potatoes.

5. Monitor Portion Sizes: Pay attention to portion sizes and consider sharing larger entrees or appetizers with dining companions to avoid overeating. If portions are generous, ask for a takeout container and save leftovers for another meal.

6. Be Mindful of Hidden Sodium: Be aware of hidden sources of sodium in restaurant meals, such as processed meats, canned

sauces, and pre-packaged ingredients. Choose dishes with fresh, whole ingredients and ask for low-sodium seasoning options when available.

7. Limit Alcohol and Beverages: Limit alcohol consumption, as alcoholic beverages can be high in calories, sugar, and sodium. Opt for water, unsweetened tea, or other low-calorie, low-sugar beverages to stay hydrated and avoid excess fluid intake.

8. Practice Portion Control: Practice portion control by sharing appetizers or desserts with others, or ordering smaller-sized portions if available. Avoid buffets or all-you-can-eat establishments, as they may encourage overeating and excessive fluid intake.

9. Stay Hydrated: Drink plenty of water before, during, and after your meal to stay hydrated and help flush out toxins from your body. Limit consumption of sugary beverages and caffeinated drinks, which can contribute to dehydration.

10. Enjoy Your Meal Mindfully: Take your time to savor and enjoy your meal mindfully, focusing on the flavors and textures of each bite. Chew slowly and stop eating when you feel satisfied, rather than overly full.

Lifestyle Advice for Dialysis Patients: Beyond the Diet

Guidelines for Physical Activity and Exercise

For individuals undergoing dialysis or managing kidney disease, physical activity and exercise can play a crucial role in improving overall health and well-being. However, it's essential to approach physical activity with caution and consideration of individual health status and medical history.

1. Consult with Healthcare Providers: Before starting any exercise program, consult with your healthcare team, including nephrologists, nurses, and physical therapists. They can assess your current health status, provide guidance on safe

exercise practices, and recommend appropriate activities based on your individual needs and limitations.

2. Start Slowly and Progress Gradually: If you're new to exercise or have been inactive for a while, start slowly with low-intensity activities and gradually increase the duration and intensity over time. Aim for at least 150 minutes of moderate-intensity aerobic exercise per week, such as walking, cycling, or swimming.

3. Choose Low-Impact Activities: Opt for low-impact exercises that are gentle on the joints and muscles, such as walking, biking, water aerobics, or Tai Chi. These activities can help improve cardiovascular fitness,

muscle strength, and flexibility without putting excessive strain on the body.

4. Include Strength Training: Incorporate strength training exercises into your routine to build and maintain muscle strength and bone density. Use light weights, resistance bands, or bodyweight exercises to target major muscle groups, such as squats, lunges, bicep curls, and chest presses.

5. Focus on Flexibility and Balance: Include flexibility and balance exercises to improve joint mobility, range of motion, and stability. Practice gentle stretching, yoga, or Pilates exercises to maintain flexibility and reduce the risk of injury.

6. Listen to Your Body: Pay attention to how your body responds to exercise and adjust your routine accordingly. If you experience pain, discomfort, dizziness, or other unusual symptoms, stop exercising and consult with your healthcare provider.

7. Stay Hydrated: Drink plenty of water before, during, and after exercise to stay hydrated and prevent dehydration. Avoid excessive fluid intake, especially if you have fluid restrictions prescribed by your healthcare team.

8. Monitor Vital Signs: Keep track of your heart rate, blood pressure, and symptoms before, during, and after exercise. Use a heart rate monitor or monitor your pulse

manually to ensure you're exercising within a safe and appropriate intensity range.

9. Be Consistent: Aim for regular, consistent exercise sessions throughout the week to maximize the benefits of physical activity. Schedule workouts at times that work best for your schedule and stick to your routine as much as possible.

10. Enjoy Variety: Keep your exercise routine interesting and enjoyable by incorporating a variety of activities and workouts. Try different types of exercise, such as walking, swimming, cycling, dancing, or gardening, to keep things fun and engaging.

Strategies for Stress Management

Managing stress is essential for overall well-being, especially for individuals undergoing dialysis or managing kidney disease.

1. Practice Relaxation Techniques: Incorporate relaxation techniques into your daily routine to reduce stress levels and promote relaxation. Techniques such as deep breathing exercises, progressive muscle relaxation, guided imagery, and meditation can help calm the mind and body.

2. Stay Active: Engage in regular physical activity and exercise to release tension, improve mood, and boost overall well-being. Aim for at least 30 minutes of

moderate-intensity exercise most days of the week, such as walking, swimming, cycling, or yoga.

3. Maintain a Healthy Lifestyle: Prioritize healthy habits such as eating a balanced diet, getting adequate sleep, and avoiding excessive alcohol and caffeine intake. These lifestyle factors can contribute to overall stress resilience and well-being.

4. Establish a Support Network: Seek support from friends, family members, support groups, or mental health professionals who can provide encouragement, understanding, and guidance during challenging times. Connecting with others who understand

your experiences can help alleviate feelings of isolation and loneliness.

5. Set Realistic Goals: Break tasks and responsibilities into manageable steps and set realistic goals for yourself. Focus on what you can control and prioritize your most important tasks, while letting go of perfectionism and unrealistic expectations.

6. Practice Time Management: Use time management techniques such as creating to-do lists, prioritizing tasks, and setting boundaries to manage your time effectively and reduce feelings of overwhelm. Delegate tasks when possible and learn to say no to additional commitments when necessary.

7. Engage in Stress-Relieving Activities: Participate in activities that bring you joy and relaxation, such as hobbies, creative pursuits, spending time in nature, or listening to music. Engaging in activities you enjoy can help distract from stressors and promote a sense of well-being.

8. Cultivate Mindfulness: Practice mindfulness techniques to increase present-moment awareness and reduce stress reactivity. Mindfulness practices such as mindful breathing, mindful eating, and body scans can help you stay grounded and centered amidst life's challenges.

9. Seek Professional Help: If stress becomes overwhelming or interferes with your daily functioning, consider seeking professional

help from a therapist, counselor, or mental health provider. Therapy can provide valuable support and guidance in developing coping skills and managing stress effectively.

10. Be Kind to Yourself: Practice self-compassion and self-care by treating yourself with kindness and understanding. Be patient with yourself during difficult times and acknowledge your efforts and accomplishments, no matter how small.

Simple and Healthful Smoothie Ideas

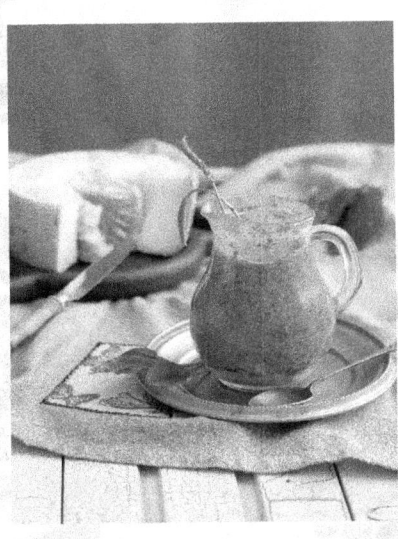

Breakfast Smoothies Low in Potassium

1. Berry Blast Smoothie:

- 1/2 cup strawberries (hulled)
- 1/2 cup blueberries
- 1/2 cup raspberries
- 1/2 cup unsweetened almond milk
- 1/2 cup plain Greek yogurt (low-potassium variety)
- 1 tablespoon honey or maple syrup (optional)

- Ice cubes (optional)

2. Green Goddess Smoothie:
- 1/2 cup spinach or kale (fresh or frozen)
- 1/2 ripe banana (frozen slices)
- 1/2 cup cucumber (peeled and chopped)
- 1/2 cup unsweetened coconut milk
- 1 tablespoon chia seeds
- 1 tablespoon almond butter (unsalted)
- Ice cubes (optional)

3. Peachy Keen Smoothie:
- 1/2 cup peaches (fresh or frozen, peeled and sliced)
- 1/2 cup pineapple (fresh or frozen, cubed)
- 1/2 cup unsweetened rice milk
- 1/2 cup plain Greek yogurt (low-potassium variety)
- 1 tablespoon ground flaxseed

- 1 teaspoon vanilla extract
- Ice cubes (optional)

4. Creamy Coconut Smoothie:
- 1/2 cup coconut milk (unsweetened)
- 1/2 cup mango (fresh or frozen, cubed)
- 1/2 cup papaya (fresh or frozen, cubed)
- 1/2 cup plain Greek yogurt (low-potassium variety)
- 1 tablespoon shredded coconut (unsweetened)
- 1 tablespoon honey or agave syrup (optional)
- Ice cubes (optional)

5. Apple Cinnamon Smoothie:
- 1/2 cup unsweetened applesauce
- 1/2 cup unsweetened almond milk
- 1/2 teaspoon ground cinnamon
- 1/4 teaspoon vanilla extract

- 1/2 cup plain Greek yogurt (low-potassium variety)
- 1 tablespoon honey or maple syrup (optional)
- Ice cubes (optional)

6. Vanilla Oatmeal Smoothie:
- 1/4 cup rolled oats (cooked and cooled)
- 1/2 ripe banana
- 1/2 cup unsweetened almond milk
- 1/2 teaspoon vanilla extract
- 1/2 cup plain Greek yogurt (low-potassium variety)
- 1 tablespoon almond butter (unsalted)
- Ice cubes (optional)

7. Tropical Paradise Smoothie:
- 1/2 cup mango (fresh or frozen, cubed)
- 1/2 cup pineapple (fresh or frozen, cubed)

-1/2 cup unsweetened coconut water

- 1/2 cup plain Greek yogurt (low-potassium variety)

- 1 tablespoon lime juice

- Ice cubes (optional)

Ideas for Nutrient-Dense Smoothies

Nutrient-dense smoothies are an excellent way to pack a variety of essential nutrients into one delicious and convenient drink.

1. Green Power Smoothie:
- Handful of spinach or kale
- 1/2 avocado
- 1/2 cucumber
- 1/2 banana
- 1/2 cup pineapple chunks
- 1 tablespoon chia seeds

- 1 tablespoon honey or maple syrup (optional)
- Water or coconut water to blend

2. Berry Antioxidant Blast:
- 1/2 cup mixed berries (such as strawberries, blueberries, raspberries)
- 1/2 cup spinach or kale
- 1/2 cup Greek yogurt (plain or vanilla)
- 1 tablespoon flaxseed or chia seeds
- 1/2 cup unsweetened almond milk or coconut water

3. Protein-Packed Peanut Butter Banana:
- 1 ripe banana
- 2 tablespoons peanut butter (unsalted)
- 1/2 cup Greek yogurt (plain or vanilla)
- 1 tablespoon honey or maple syrup (optional)

- 1/2 cup unsweetened almond milk or dairy milk
- Handful of spinach (optional for added nutrients)

4. Creamy Coconut Mango Smoothie:
- 1/2 cup mango chunks (fresh or frozen)
- 1/2 cup coconut milk (canned or homemade)
- 1/2 cup Greek yogurt (plain or vanilla)
- 1 tablespoon shredded coconut (unsweetened)
- 1 tablespoon chia seeds or hemp seeds
- Ice cubes (optional)

5. Banana Almond Butter Oatmeal Smoothie:
- 1 ripe banana
- 2 tablespoons almond butter (unsalted)

- 1/4 cup rolled oats
- 1/2 cup Greek yogurt (plain or vanilla)
- 1 tablespoon honey or maple syrup (optional)
- 1/2 teaspoon cinnamon
- 1/2 cup unsweetened almond milk or dairy milk

6. Tropical Turmeric Smoothie:
- 1/2 cup pineapple chunks
- 1/2 cup mango chunks
- 1/2 banana
- 1/2 teaspoon ground turmeric
- 1/2 teaspoon fresh grated ginger
- 1/2 cup Greek yogurt (plain or vanilla)
- 1 tablespoon honey or maple syrup (optional)
- Water or coconut water to blend

7. Chocolate Avocado Protein Smoothie:

- 1/2 ripe avocado
- 1 tablespoon cocoa powder (unsweetened)
- 1 scoop chocolate protein powder
- 1/2 cup Greek yogurt (plain or chocolate)
- 1 tablespoon honey or maple syrup (optional)
- 1/2 cup unsweetened almond milk or dairy milk

Recipes for Breakfast Bowls for Patients on Dialysis

1. Berry Breakfast Bowl:
- 1/2 cup cooked quinoa or oatmeal
- 1/2 cup mixed berries (such as strawberries, blueberries, raspberries)

- 1 tablespoon chopped nuts (almonds, walnuts, or pecans)
- 1 tablespoon seeds (chia seeds, hemp seeds, or flaxseeds)
- 1/4 cup Greek yogurt (low-potassium variety)
- 1 teaspoon honey or maple syrup (optional)

2. Tropical Smoothie Bowl:
- 1/2 cup Greek yogurt (low-potassium variety)
- 1/2 banana (sliced)
- 1/2 cup mango chunks (fresh or frozen)
- 1/4 cup pineapple chunks (fresh or frozen)
- 1 tablespoon shredded coconut (unsweetened)
- 1 tablespoon chopped nuts or seeds (optional)

- 1 teaspoon honey or agave syrup (optional)

3. Nutty Banana Breakfast Bowl:
- 1/2 cup cooked quinoa or oatmeal
- 1/2 banana (sliced)
- 1 tablespoon almond butter (unsalted)
- 1 tablespoon chopped nuts (such as almonds or walnuts)
- 1 tablespoon seeds (chia seeds, hemp seeds, or flaxseeds)
- Dash of cinnamon
- 1 teaspoon honey or maple syrup (optional)

4. Apple Cinnamon Breakfast Bowl:
- 1/2 cup cooked quinoa or oatmeal
- 1/2 apple (diced)
- 1 tablespoon chopped nuts (such as almonds or pecans)

- 1 tablespoon dried cranberries or raisins
- Dash of cinnamon
- 1/4 cup Greek yogurt (low-potassium variety)
- 1 teaspoon honey or maple syrup (optional)

5. Protein-Packed Breakfast Bowl:
- 1/2 cup cooked quinoa or brown rice
- 1/4 cup black beans (canned, rinsed, and drained)
- 1/4 avocado (sliced)
- 1/2 cup diced tomatoes
- 1 tablespoon chopped cilantro
- 1 tablespoon salsa (low-sodium)
- 1 tablespoon shredded cheese (low-sodium)
- Poached or boiled egg (optional)

6. Greek Yogurt Parfait Bowl:
- 1/2 cup Greek yogurt (low-potassium variety)
- 1/4 cup granola (low-sodium and low-potassium)
- 1/2 cup mixed berries (such as strawberries, blueberries)
- 1 tablespoon chopped nuts (such as almonds or walnuts)
- 1 teaspoon honey or maple syrup (optional)

7. Savory Breakfast Bowl:
- 1/2 cup cooked quinoa or brown rice
- Sautéed vegetables (such as spinach, bell peppers, onions)
- 1/4 cup cooked lentils or chickpeas
- 1/4 avocado (sliced)
- Poached or boiled egg

- Fresh herbs (such as parsley or cilantro)
- Dash of hot sauce or salsa (low-sodium)

Conclusion

Summary of Important Ideas

Dietary Considerations: Follow a kidney-friendly diet that is low in sodium, potassium, and phosphorus. Choose nutrient-dense foods such as fruits, vegetables, lean proteins, and whole grains. Be mindful of portion sizes and avoid processed or high-potassium foods.

Meal Planning: Plan balanced meals and snacks that meet your nutritional needs while adhering to dietary restrictions. Consult with a dietitian to develop personalized meal plans and learn strategies for managing dietary limitations effectively.

Smoothies and Breakfast Bowls: Incorporate nutrient-dense smoothies and breakfast bowls into your diet for convenient and delicious meal options. Choose ingredients that are low in potassium and phosphorus, such as berries, Greek yogurt, nuts, seeds, and whole grains.

Physical Activity: Engage in regular physical activity and exercise to improve cardiovascular health, muscle strength, and overall well-being. Choose low-impact activities such as walking, swimming, or cycling and consult with healthcare providers before starting an exercise program.

Stress Management: Practice stress management techniques such as relaxation exercises, mindfulness, and staying active to reduce stress levels and promote emotional well-being. Seek support from healthcare providers, family members, or support groups when needed.

Hydration: Stay hydrated by drinking plenty of water throughout the day, but be mindful of fluid restrictions prescribed by healthcare providers. Limit consumption of sugary beverages, caffeine, and alcohol, which can contribute to dehydration.

Medication Management: Take medications as prescribed by healthcare providers and attend regular appointments to monitor kidney function, manage symptoms, and adjust treatment plans as needed.

Self-Care: Prioritize self-care and well-being by getting adequate rest, managing stress, and engaging in activities that bring joy and relaxation. Practice self-compassion and seek support from others when facing challenges related to kidney disease and dialysis.

Sources of Additional Information

For additional information on managing kidney disease and dialysis, as well as related topics such as nutrition, exercise, and stress management, consider exploring reputable sources such as:

The NKF is a leading organization dedicated to raising awareness, providing education, and supporting individuals affected by kidney disease. Their website offers a wealth of resources, including educational materials, patient resources, and information on treatment options.

The AKF is another valuable resource for individuals with kidney disease, offering educational programs, financial assistance, and advocacy initiatives. Their website provides information on kidney health, dialysis, transplantation, and living with kidney disease.

The CDC offers information and resources on kidney disease prevention, risk factors, and management. Their website includes educational materials, statistics, and guidelines for healthcare providers and patients.

National Institute of Diabetes and Digestive and Kidney Diseases (NIDDK): NIDDK, part of the National Institutes of Health (NIH), conducts research and provides information on various kidney-related conditions, including kidney disease, dialysis, and transplantation. Their website offers resources for patients, healthcare professionals, and researchers.

Renal Support Network (RSN): RSN is a patient-led organization that provides support, education, and advocacy for individuals affected by kidney disease. Their website features patient stories, educational materials, and resources for coping with kidney disease and dialysis.

Davita Kidney Care is a leading provider of kidney care services, including dialysis treatment and education. Their website offers educational articles, recipes, and resources for patients living with kidney disease and undergoing dialysis.

KidneyBuzz is an online platform that provides information, support, and resources for individuals living with kidney disease. Their website features articles, videos, and community forums where patients can connect and share experiences.

Consider reading books and publications authored by healthcare professionals, dietitians, and individuals living with kidney disease. Look for titles on topics [1]such as

---
[1]

renal nutrition, dialysis management, and coping with kidney disease.

Joining support groups and community organizations for individuals with kidney disease can provide valuable support, information, and encouragement. Look for local or online groups where you can connect with others facing similar challenges.

Finally, don't hesitate to reach out to your healthcare providers, including nephrologists, dietitians, nurses, and social workers, for personalized information and guidance on managing kidney disease and dialysis. They can offer tailored advice, answer questions, and provide support throughout your journey.

Request for Review

Greetings, Reader

We are appreciative that you are reading "Kidney Dialysis Diet Cookbook for Seniors" written by Mike J. Clack. We really hope that the knowledge and perspectives offered in this book were beneficial to you.

Your opinions are valuable to us. We respectfully request that you consider providing a review if you found this book to be informative and enjoyable to read. By reading your review, other readers will be able to learn more about this book and decide whether it's the perfect choice for them.

Please think about discussing the following when you write your review:

What you found most enjoyable about the book; How it improved your knowledge of the subject; Any particular advice or suggestions you found especially helpful; and Whether or not you would suggest this book to others, along with your reasons.

Reviews may be left on websites like Amazon.com.

In addition to assisting the author, your review will assist other readers in making well-informed judgements on whether or not to read this book.

Once again, I would like to thank you for reading "Kidney Dialysis Diet Cookbook for Seniors". We are grateful for your support and hope the material will continue to be useful to you.

Warm regards,

www.ingramcontent.com/pod-product-compliance
Lightning Source LLC
Chambersburg PA
CBHW052205220526
45471CB00004B/1825